How I Restore My Brain Abilities

The Right Way and Legally

DR. ANDREA SCARSI

DEDICATED

I am trying to remember who now

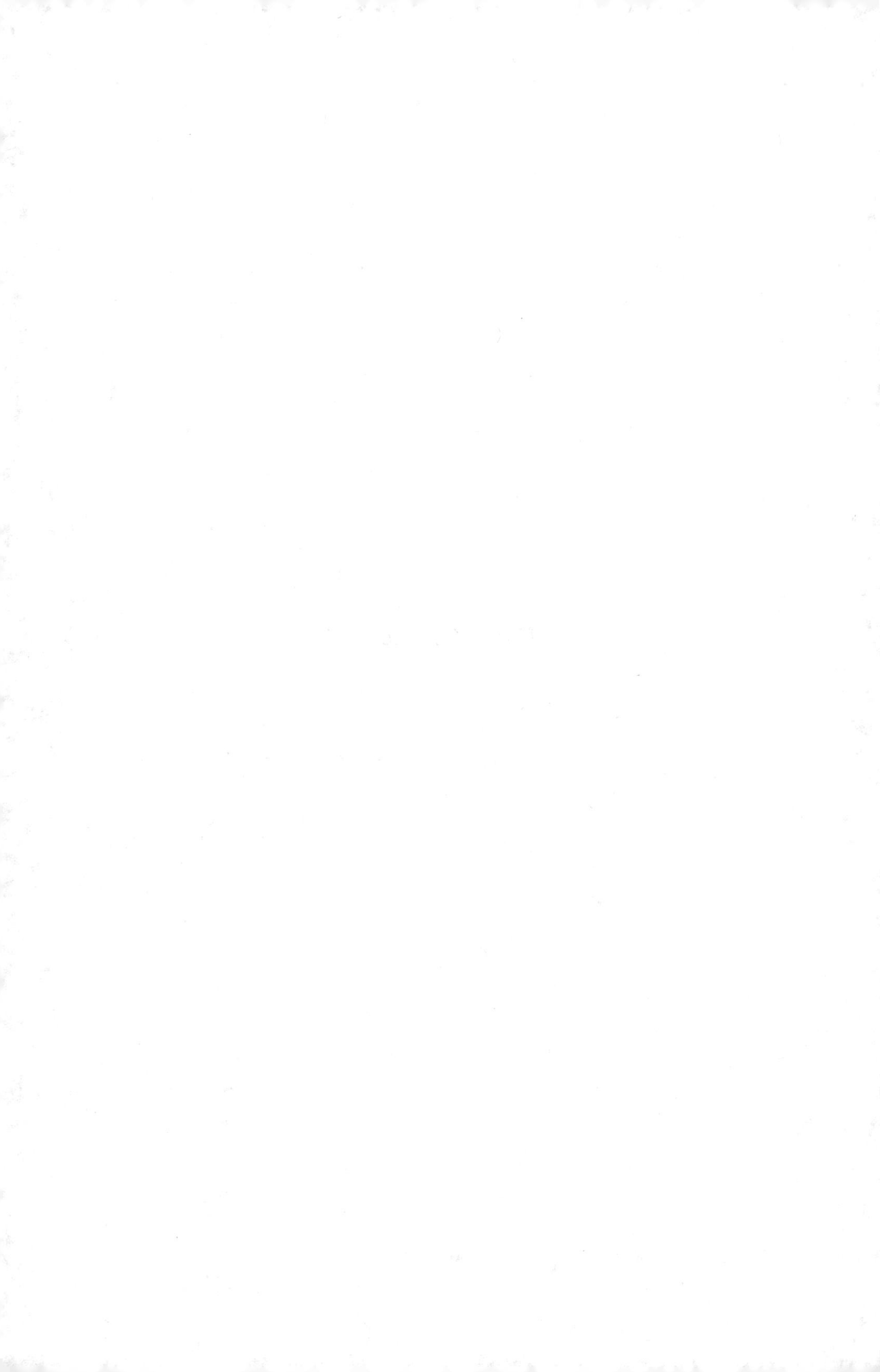

INDEX

Dr. ANDREA SCARSI

ACKNOWLEDGMENTS

I thank those who give me daily examples of brilliance, drowsiness, slowness, and emptiness. Now, I remember that I dedicate this book to them.

I thank my dear friend Dr. Sevaram Sharma, head of geriatrics at a German geriatric rehabilitation clinic, for the precious information he provided me while walking along the seashore without stopping.

I am deeply indebted to Mother Nature for her boundless generosity. She has provided me with everything I need, even when I have forgotten that I owe my existence to her. Her role in fostering the awareness of my forgetfulness is a testament to her profound influence on my life and work.

NOTE OF THE AUTHOR

The Author strived to be accurate and complete when creating this book. Nevertheless, he affirms that the contents expressed in it are solely the result of his knowledge, experience, and competence in the considered discipline and does not guarantee and declare at any time that these are absolute and unequivocal.

While he made all attempts to verify the information in this publication, he assumes no responsibility for errors, omissions, different interpretations, or experimentations of the subject matter herein.

Any perceived slights of specific persons, peoples, companies, or organizations are unintentional.

As one expects, self-help books and manuals do not guarantee results or income. Readers must rely on their judgment about any single circumstance and act accordingly.

This book does not pretend to be an official medical, dietetic, psychological, religious, legal, commercial, accounting, or financial professional source. The Readers must seek the services of competent professionals in all the abovementioned fields.

Enjoy your practice.

Dr. ANDREA SCARSI

DESCRIPTION

Suppose you are looking to learn everything there is to know about how to restore your brain's capabilities. In that case, this is the correct information for you and perhaps even the most critical information you will ever read, simply because all the new discoveries on the subject have been proven and reported in this fantastic new book titled, How I Restore My Brain Abilities.

The book covers almost every piece of news anyone could want to know about the subject. Imagine restoring your brain's capabilities quickly—because those who start are already halfway there—without any sense of frustration and, above all, without wasting time on research, consultations, and field tests—from the comfort of your home.

This is fantastic, and, in fact, it is. Yes, you can have a better life; you can return to the capabilities of your youth and even improve them. It is definitely possible; you just need to know how. The how is explained in detail in this new, incredible book, written to help you make this dream of yours come true, to help you restore your brain capacity.

Assimilate what is suggested; root your decision to do it; practice the exercises and strategies indicated; adjust your diet; organize your ideas; know what to do and not to do; play; stimulate your senses; renew your environment; exercise; relax, meditate, discover who you are. Invest in restoring your brain capacity; it is easy, and you deserve the satisfaction of enjoying all your days and everything life offers you.

This is the teaching.

INTRODUCTION

Years ago, I had a disturbing and terrible situation with my memory. Every day, I had to force myself to remember where I had put my house or car keys, my wallet, my sunglasses, and the names of people and things in general, and the problem not only did not disappear but persisted. In fact, it got worse month after month. It was as if my brain had suddenly aged and continued to age.

I then noticed something even more worrying, at least for me, who is still young: I was no longer as fast at processing information as I had been a few years earlier; I could no longer do calculations beyond two digits, my thinking was slow, and I was losing my mental agility. It was then that I decided to do something about it. Nothing was physically wrong with my brain, but something was no longer working as it should or was missing.

After thinking about it long and hard, of course, I concluded that I needed a new lifestyle regimen adequate to restore my brain capacity once again. If you can apply strategies to strengthen the body, you can also do something to optimize the brain.

I created a personal training regimen to improve my memory and thinking ability. I began seriously researching the basic principles of brain enhancement and increasing its neurological capacity for synthesis.

Little by little, my functionality improved; I was no longer forgetful and felt that my gray cells had regained youthful agility. The brain's potential has nothing to do with age; if I know how and what to do, I can easily keep it healthy as I grow older.

This brain training regimen is one of my most significant discoveries, and this book aims to share precisely how I regained, with great satisfaction, the brain agility, creativity, and ability to remember anything instantly.

I did not pay attention to these abilities in my youth; I took them for granted, and it is essential to keep them active.

The day I decided to improve my memory and restore my brain's capacity was a great day of rebirth. No more anxiety or worry; in fact, there are simple and natural methods of brain optimization without the use of drugs, medications, or expensive therapies.

THE MULTIPLE STRATEGIES

Let me make one thing clear right away: if I said there was only one sure way to restore brain capacity, I would be lying because, in fact, my human brain can be strengthened and stimulated in so many ways that it is tough to choose or settle on a single strategy; there are simply so many, they are all good, and therefore I use all or almost all of them and I indicate them in the first part of the book, to subsequently address the specific foods that I have integrated into my diet to adequately nourish my synapses and improve the functionality of my brain in general.

Important Note: Some strategies require more work than others. Therefore, I choose those feasible in the first days and weeks of practice and feel free to add others as and when I see fit.

I LISTEN TO MUSIC

Music is one of the world's oldest and most effective therapeutic modalities. It is and has been used for many things: to elevate, calm, and stabilize moods, to put babies to sleep, and to increase the IQ of unborn babies. For some time, and still in some quarters, it was believed that listening to classical music could do this. However, as I focus on restoring my adult brainpower, here is how music helps me achieve this goal.

1. Music has been and is widely used as a supportive treatment for anxiety disorders. If I feel anxious or agitated most of the time due to stress at work or home, I listen to music, which helps me manage what I am feeling at that moment. Music does not reshape the external situation, whatever it is; it does not calm the person yelling at me, but it helps me stay sane, even though I have to deal with work, traffic, and relationship issues daily. The trick is to always allow myself to recover from stress. Stressors are a part of life; I can only disconnect from them occasionally to take care of myself mentally and physically.

2. Established studies and popular wisdom show that listening to certain music, such as relaxing music, can lower high blood pressure and benefit those suffering from dementia. University studies have also shown that music can even help premature babies gain more weight in a shorter period than

those without music therapy. I can only imagine how powerful the effect of musical vibration is on the human body, if it can even encourage tissue growth and weight gain.

3. Listening to music and playing musical instruments has increased vital brain areas, such as the corpus callosum, responsible for connecting the two cerebral hemispheres. It has also been shown that playing musical instruments increases the size of the motor cortex of the brain precisely because it is an activity that requires not only knowledge of music theory but also dexterity and manual skill when manipulating the instrument. Furthermore, recent brain tomography technology indicates that both my lobes light up when listening to music. At the same time, when I hear songs, I tend to give more importance to meanings, lighting up only the lobe that manages logic.

4. Playing music helps me continuously improve spatial skills, so I don't worry if I can't play decently now because my brain ensures I can play well when I learn a new instrument. I choose a musical instrument I like to play at home and try to understand it myself. I can also hire a teacher if that's what I want. The important thing here is that I can learn something new, play a musical instrument, and listen to music simultaneously.

You can listen to music, songs, and mantras on my YouTube cannel playlist.

I KEEP A JOURNAL

Recent studies have shown that regularly keeping a journal is effective in restoring my thinking skills and helps me manage stress. Journaling is great if my thinking is disorganized and I have trouble piecing together ideas and what I need to do to achieve them.

Journaling is different from writing a to-do list. My journal writing focuses on my current experiences and self-expression. I get a good notebook or diary and start writing.

Sometimes, I prefer to use my computer or my phone or start my own blog; I am free to switch between them and do as I wish, but when I feel like my thoughts are my own, and I enjoy the solitude and peace that a regular journal provides, then I take out a notebook and continue on paper.

It is easy to start a journal and just write. I do not focus on making my handwriting extremely beautiful or legible. I don't focus on the look but on the idea and getting my emotions and ideas onto paper or a keyboard.

Keeping a journal is all mine and all for me. It's something I enjoy. Writing in my journal is fun and rewarding, but I don't have to do it daily if I'm bored or feel obligated. Sure, some initiative is essential when I'm trying to accomplish something, but at the same time, if I feel horrible when I try to write, that's not the best option for me right now. But if journaling or writing two things brings me pleasure and fun, I'll continue because I know it helps restore my brain's capacity.

Want an example of a journal? See my book, 21 Days.

I BUILD MY MIND MAPS

Mind maps, or groups of interconnected ideas, are graphic representations of the organization of my thoughts when I reflect on a project and reproduce my brain's neural network. They stimulate my visual memory capacity and increase my ability to remember concepts by structuring them in mental hierarchy relationships, associating them, and highlighting their connections and concatenations.

They stimulate my creativity and focus because I develop them in an absolutely personal way, with my own words, unique and colorful that make them pleasant and leave room for new associations, possible integrations, and intuitions by activating my right cerebral hemisphere, the seat of my functions of creativity, memory, and mental association.

Even though excellent software programs allow me to create my mind maps on a computer, tablet, or cell phone, I prefer to build them on paper or a large blackboard. So, I bought a reasonably large sketchbook with lots of paper and beautiful colored markers that give me a more toned experience, more freedom of movement, and more breadth of vision.

I use my mind maps both for my personal use and for my work. Even if those maps look like ramifications of extravagant and uncertain ideas and words, they are only like that because they are my mind maps and personal expressions that give meaning to me, who created them. When I share them, friends and colleagues only sometimes understand them immediately because everyone thinks in their own way, and what makes perfect sense to me can be confusing and completely baffling to the person on the other side of the table.

When I create my mind map, I do the following.

1. I just think of one thing I want to plan or track. It can be a story I have always wanted to write, a trip I have always wanted to take, or a plan to reach a financial goal in several years. They are all fine; any idea of what I want to do is a viable starting point.

2. I break the idea into two or three big ideas. For example, I aspire to achieve a specific economic condition. In that case, the big ideas I draw in my one-word map include selling great, unique products that people love, producing those great products, and marketing those great products. I extend my mind map indefinitely by adding more and more ideas related to the starting central idea.

3. After I have my big ideas down, I stop and expand them. I start creating the first branches of my basic big idea, and after the first level of expansion, I start making more branches in my mind map. If one idea leads to another, I immediately connect those two ideas. Ultimately, I have a mind map that accurately reflects the nerve cells in my brain. I use appropriate spacing and long, curved lines that clearly separate the big groups of ideas from each other. If one page isn't enough for me, I flip to the next page, and that's the beauty of having a sketchbook with lots of paper.

PS: These mind maps also reflect my work in Network Marketing. I am at the center, and the lines of collaboration and clientele develop around me. Do you want to know more about Network Marketing?

I ENJOY POWER NAPS

Rest is essential to my health, although some feel perfectly rested after only 4 or 5 hours of sleep daily. I guess that's true, but sticking to this type of sleep schedule damages my brain's ability to recall and retain memories, for example, and my overall health.

Getting too little sleep each night can actually increase the risk of severe health problems. Sleep is essential to the human body, so my current strategy focuses on rest, even if only for short periods.

When I can squeeze in a thirty-minute break in the middle of the day, I've done a great thing. If I can only nap for 15 minutes, that's fine too.

The benefits of power naps add up over a week, and my entire body, including my brain, appreciates that I'm setting aside even short periods for recovery.

When I have memory problems, I am often physically healthy and fit but simply exhausted and fatigued from overwork. Work is important because it gives me direction and stabilizes my finances. Still, work should never cause me mental and physical discomfort, and when it does, I immediately reevaluate my work style and general working conditions.

Sleep is also essential because we dream. If you are interested in dreams, see my book A Brief History of Dreams.

I KEEP MY BLOOD PRESSURE IN ORDER

Recent studies have shown that older adults with high blood pressure are at risk of lower cognitive performance than people who manage their condition with medications or natural blood pressure control methods such as meditation and diet changes.

They also showed that suffering from hypertension between the ages of twenty and thirty is not a particularly good thing because, over time, the effects on cognitive performance add up. Ultimately, the risk of a marked decrease in brain function is noticeable with advancing age. For this reason, I always keep my blood pressure at optimal levels.

I am an example of this. My GP, at a certain point in my life, gives me an ultimatum: "Either you take the pill for blood pressure, or I will stop you from flying." At that time, I flew often, and clearly, I gave in to the blackmail.

A few years later, however, when a friend explained to me the influence of weight on this pathology, I decided to get myself back in order by starting a new nutritional path, accompanied by a coach and using the products of the Herbalife company.

We did the nutritional analysis. I started with a balanced breakfast, and immediately, the weight began to drop. I felt better, more energetic, and alert. The coach was fundamental, always present, and gave me all the support I needed.

In a month and a half, I lost 5 kilos and two sizes, and the doctor made me stop taking the pill! I continued, and my life always returned to fluid, lively, slim, and lucid. In 7 months, I lost 20 kilos, which I have not regained, like the pill, and I am so happy, to the point of becoming an Independent Herbalife Distributor myself.

I MEDITATE

Meditation combines physical and mental relaxation to achieve a state of complete physical calm and mental clarity. In general, meditation has no religious ties, although, in popular culture, it is strongly associated with Eastern spiritual practices. Meditation is used by Buddhists and Hindus, but that doesn't mean I have to be a Buddhist monk before I can meditate. Meditation is for everyone, and especially for me.

Meditation offers me the following benefits.

1. It lowers my anxiety levels and calms my nerves.

2. It improves my breathing pattern, which, in turn, has a positive effect on my thought process.

3. It lowers my blood pressure and improves my stress and pain management.

4. It clears my mind of cobwebs when I need to be creative and spontaneous.

For example, when I feel stiff and bored before any public performance, such as a conference or presentation to my boss and colleagues, I meditate to improve how I process and relate information to others.

Meditation is easy. Just download a good book on meditation from Amazon, such as mine, The Secret of Meditation, and apply the suggestions, at first only for a few minutes each day.

The results always surprise me. I don't expect miracles, but I don't give up and follow my progress, which improves daily, giving my brain time to adapt to my new activities. My brain wants to improve at what it does best, which is out of the question.

FIT BODY FIT BRAIN

I had the wrong idea that physical exercise only benefits my muscles, bones, and joints and does not affect my brain. That is not true. Even though I knew the proverb, I was wrong knowing I was wrong. According to established medical science and current research in this area, exercise has a very beneficial effect on my brain.

In fact, exercise has been proven to be an efficient and natural way to improve the mind's ability to process information quickly. This ability is the solid foundation of a restored mind, regardless of what I want to achieve, such as crunching numbers faster or maximizing my creativity.

Sometimes, I fall into the trap of using food to stimulate my mind and creative flow. This is not good for my body because it clogs up, and a practice that gives in to food cravings is a clear sign that I am associating food with good feelings and ideas. Next time I need inspiration before I give in to the habit of reaching for a bag of chips and a sugary drink, I will try some form of workout, perhaps with barbells.

Working out does not mean I must join a fitness gym and lift hefty weights like professionals or aspiring ones. My best workouts are fun because I choose the activity that I like at the moment and can also vary from time to time. Physical fitness does not need to be excruciating; I enjoy doing it in the first place, and I do not need to force myself to start and complete.

Here are some activities that give me a good workout; I choose one, two, or as many as I want, depending on where I am, but only fun and exciting. I enjoy walking, running, swimming, cycling, jogging, yoga - especially Sun Salutation, Surya Namaskara, watching the sun of course - beach tennis, skiing, skating, Nordic walking, lifting light weights, dancing, belly dancing, aerobics, sex, mixed martial arts, karate, judo, taichi, taekwondo, boxing, kickboxing, kayaking, sailing, archery, climbing, skydiving and singing.

These are just a few of the most common sports or physical activities I practice every day worldwide. There are as many physical activities as days in the year, and maybe even more. So, I find what my body craves and get my brain and heart pumping hard.

I don't need to slow down because I'm getting older, but on the contrary, taking it easy makes me rusty. A healthy body leads to a healthier mind, regardless of my age.

I STIMULATE MY MIND WITH GAMES

When I am forced to look at the same four walls day in and day out, I am at high risk for depression and a myriad of other psychological problems because I am deprived of the mental stimulation that keeps my mind in tip-top shape. Because my human brain has evolved to handle so much stimulation, it actually degenerates if it is not stimulated. My brain is a muscle; if I do not use my muscles, they decay and become brittle and weak. I do not want to weaken one of the most essential organs in my body, my power plant.

One of the most accessible ways to stimulate my mind is through games, and I am never too old for games. Here is the thing: I do not stop enjoying games because I have reached a certain age. I do not think that as an adult, I should only focus on serious, adult things; that is not the case, and it is not even possible; I have been who I have been since I was born, I have developed, but I am still the same, I like the same things, and I have the same impulses as always. I will change when everything changes.

Going back to before, the truth is that if I want to focus on adult responsibilities and the critical issues of a certain age, I must keep my brain stimulated and ready for action. The easiest way to do this is to play. Like when I was a child. Games that require other players are great, such as card games and board games, to kill two birds with one stone because social interaction is also essential for brain recovery. Still, when I cannot invite friends or colleagues to play such games daily, the best thing is computer games, cell phones, or PlayStation.

I have such equipment at home or in my pocket in this historical period. It does not matter what game console or platform I use at home or with me; the important thing is to play. I play for one or two hours a day during leisure moments and in the intervals between one situation and another. I also avoid exaggerating. Playing all day or more than six hours at a time is too much for my mind and health.

I like playing with Tarot and Crystals. See My books: Tarot Reading and Welcome to Atlantis.

I READ MORE BOOKS

Despite the many changes in the way I communicate with people and friends in today's world, I still find a space in my daily routine to read books.

I no longer have to buy printed books because I no longer need to do so with my tablet, cell phone, and e-reader. I also believe that this will save forests, and I will also avoid breathing in dust and mites.

I read to stimulate my mind.

In fact, a good read leaves a lasting mental impression on me because it stimulates both the rational side of my brain, which follows the story's unfolding, and the intuitive side, which builds images that depict the story, the places, and the characters.

It also stimulates my emotions to participate in the events. Even a good movie does that, but it already gives me scenarios and does not allow me to use my imagination and visualization skills.

When I find a talented author, the book completely takes me and stimulates all my senses and imagination, sending my brain into sensory saturation. This produces immense benefits and happily increases my mental ability.

If I haven't picked up a good book for a while and most of the things I read are on the Internet or just for work, I miss something and desire to find an interesting read. Now, with self-publishing, the reading possibilities are endless. Books or ebooks, it's entirely up to me what to read; I just have to start doing it again.

Do you like reading? Please read all my other books, too.

I LEARN SOMETHING NEW

Psychologists and therapists in related fields agree that continuous learning is essential to keeping my mind strong. Learning something new occasionally is an excellent way to keep my brain young and sharp. I don't have to know anything significant at first; I just start by cultivating the habit of looking for new things to learn so that I can restore my brain power. Here are some great examples to begin with.

1. I learn to play a new musical instrument
2. I take a new route to work.
3. I discover a new route when I get home.
4. I build a model train, airplane, or boat.
5. I draw with my non-dominant hand.
6. I learn a new foreign language.
7. I volunteer in a position that requires frequent speaking and conveying information to people of different ages and walks of life.

For example, as an information desk assistant at the town library, even though I know little about indexing systems and how libraries work, I desire to learn something new that will allow me to move forward, take the plunge, and reap the benefits I want.

I currently have a new job as a holistic coach.

SOCIALIZING MAKES MY BRAIN HAPPIER AND HEALTHIER

These days, my hectic lifestyle often prevents me from meeting and genuinely connecting with other people. The lack of social interaction is one of the reasons I feel tired, burned out, and uninspired at home and work. I am a social being.

I need to interact with others because I deny myself one of my most basic structural units if I don't. Socializing also has two main benefits.

1. Regular interaction challenges and stimulates my brain. Regular stimulation encourages the formation of new neural connections. Simply put, if I give my brain enough stimulation, it has a reason to grow and expand its neural network.

2. Recent research has shown that if I don't socialize regularly, I am at a higher risk for worrying, depression, and other mental illnesses than those who make sure to socialize regularly.

Interacting with people I want to be with also helps me manage stress from home or work. I deserve to disconnect from sources of stress just as much as anyone else, so there is really no reason why I can't disconnect, even temporarily, from any sources of personal stress.

I may not be able to completely disengage from these sources of stress, but I can undoubtedly separate myself from them long enough to de-stress. I need to stay mentally healthy if I want my brain to repair itself.

I am currently socializing on a variety of topics on social media.

I WEAVE STORIES IN MY MIND

I have already experienced how easy it is to create my own mind maps on paper or in a sketchbook. I like that approach to resetting the structure of my brain, and it is nice to express my ideas in that way. Weaving stories is another similar exercise, but it is a little more complex, and I love it.

This brain exercise is simple: When I wake up in the morning, instead of running to the bathroom to brush my teeth, I sit on the edge of the bed and collect my thoughts. At first, it took a bit of effort and practice to get used to it, but in the end, I got the hang of it, and now I find it very fun.

After collecting my thoughts, I describe how I feel and how the environment appears. I open the window and look out. What do I see? And I describe what I see. Do I like looking out, or do I not like what I see? And why? And I spin a story about why I like or dislike what I see or am doing.

The trick is to become as observant as possible and notice things you usually overlook because you take them for granted. This is especially effective when my thinking is so slow that I have trouble paying attention at work or school.

Of course, I don't want to worry too much because this kind of mental state is usually just the result of understimulation and fatigue. If I know I'm overworked, I better address that first, or exercises like this won't work very well.

Here's another critical point to be aware of and keep in mind. If a particular approach isn't working for me, other factors at work or at home are likely preventing me from succeeding with that specific approach. In this case, it is really best for me to take a step back and evaluate what is preventing me from achieving what I want and, once identified, address the problem before moving on to the main goal, which is to take a favorable approach to restore my brain capacity.

This sub-step is essential to my success because if I do not remove the obstacles to my main goal, I will probably fail and feel even more frustrated than I was initially.

Now, I return to storytelling, and these are some suggestions I give myself to get started.

1. I make a game of the exercise. I look for new ways to describe everyday objects and situations. I challenge my brain to come up with strange and exotic ways to explain what I see in front of me. I step outside my usual way of seeing the world and am often surprised by how interesting it is.

2. I pay attention to all my senses. I am eye-centric, like most people, but this can be debilitating if I focus only on what I see when I have other senses equally effective at receiving sensory input. So, I notice all my senses when weaving a story based on my daily experience.

If I am in an exciting situation, I describe it in terms of what I see, hear, smell, and feel on my skin and taste in my mouth, as well as the thoughts that are going through my mind, my perception of external and internal space, the feelings I experience, and my connection to the universal.

By challenging my brain this way, I help it revive its natural creativity, which is helpful in many life situations, not just during artistic activities.

Creativity and logical thinking need to meet whenever I am solving something. My mental processing is much more effective when logic and creativity interact on everything from problems to challenges to planning a vacation.

3. When I want, I write the whole story in my journal, and

that's where I get back to the strategy I've already recommended to myself to carry out for the well-being and longevity of my brain. As already seen, writing in the journal is quite simple once I start, and sometimes, creating my story is better when I write it down rather than just thinking about it.

Writing helps me distill and refine my ideas, which is fantastic when I need to organize them. I don't need an expert to read my journal; I just need to write, write, and write more, and my style visibly improves over time.

4. Once I have mastered describing everyday objects and experiences, I challenge myself further by avoiding my usual ways of expressing things and developing new terminology and syntactic structures. Language has infinite permutations, and I do not limit myself to just one way of describing life.

GETTING MOVED

If I feel sad and uninspired at home or at work for no particular reason and think something is depressing me, before I worry that I'm losing control of the situation, I think about the fact that my brain probably just wants some new stimulation and some form of change in my environment. I introduce a change or two or three to my immediate environment, and my brain immediately appreciates the change.

If I immerse myself in an environment that doesn't change for too long, my natural creativity grinds to a halt. Here are some ways I get back in the saddle and keep my mind sharp and alert.

1. I create a garden in my backyard, which can also be a zen garden or a pond with aquatic plants. Designing my dream garden, choosing the plants and flowers, and making it a reality is good for my brain, entire body, and spirit. I shape and care for it daily, which is also a great exercise. It is just what experts recommend to restore the brain's capacity.

By creating a garden, I kill two birds with one stone again: I change my environment and exercise daily without going to the gym or a dance class.

2. I redesign my living room, bedroom, and study. Of course, there are always things I would like to change in my living spaces at home. I choose a manageable room or space and

consider changing it to fit my current preferences.

3. If the redesign is too complicated or expensive, I buy new works of art to put in the living room, kitchen, or bedroom or framed prints I can find online or at some private exhibition in the city. Often, decorating is just as good for me as redesigning an entire space. Sometimes, I prefer bonsai or some beautiful ornamental plants in pots to prints or paintings. I stick to what works for me, what I like, and what satisfies my aesthetic tastes. I always ensure that what I add to my living space improves the mood, the overall perspective of the space I have modified, and the resulting internal reflection. Being satisfied with my effort is part of the exercise of resetting my brain.

Want to tidy up your home? Check out my book, Home Sweet Home Staging.

I STIMULATE MY SENSES

Like most people, I am also eye-centric and use my eyes mainly to get information from my surroundings. That is fine, but it does not mean I must neglect all my other senses.

If I want my mind to be strong and agile, it must constantly receive stimulation from all my senses. It is not enough for me to smell, hear, taste, and feel things randomly throughout the day; I also have to be aware of them, present, able to catalog them, and challenged by my senses to create new experiences for myself.

I do this quite often, and my brain starts making new neural connections because it receives new and unique sensory input. I continue to surprise it, so it has a reason to stay agile as it ages.

Here are some techniques I practice to get started.

1. I visit a flower shop and smell the flowers. I describe the flowers and the flower shop, in general, using only my nose. In this situation, my nose acts as my eyes, so to speak, but I don't rely on them for information; I smell the air for answers.

2. I live in a relatively active neighborhood and sit in front of my house with my eyes closed. This time, I challenged my sense of hearing. I listen to my surroundings and paint a picture in my mind. What do I understand just by listening to my surroundings? What is happening right now by listening to my immediate environment? Can I tell what is happening before me, even if my eyes are closed? Yes, I can; what I get from it is

always true.

After this little exercise, I take out my journal and start writing about my experience. This is a great way to stimulate my senses and creative and logical centers.

3. Now, I stimulate my sense of touch, which is relatively easy. I open my closet and touch the different fabrics of my clothes. I describe each fabric as it touches my skin. I compare the tactile sensation of when I feel something with my hands to the sensation of when I touch it with my cheek. There are marked differences that I write in my diary.

4. As for my sense of taste, I usually only taste what I really like to eat, and I rarely go near unfamiliar foods, like miso soup, for example. Therefore, when grocery shopping, I always buy food products that are not included in my usual shopping list and my diet. I purchase something exotic and different to stimulate my accustomed and bored taste buds.

When I taste something new, I savor it like professional tasters do, with extreme attention and presence, biting only small amounts of food and moving it around my mouth to expose my entire tongue like tasting wine. Each part of the tongue detects a specific taste: bitter, sweet, salty, sour, and four tactile sensations that are spicy, astringent, texture, and temperature. Moving the food in the mouth allows the tongue and palate to thoroughly examine its tastes and aspects. Then, as usual, I write my experience in my diary.

5. My eyes, now, although abused by looking at the computer and cell phone all day, do not mean that they have received a good dose of stimuli. To stimulate my eyes, I visit colorful places, natural and natural, such as a fabric house or a flower shop. I use only my eyes to remember and describe what surrounds me this time. When the first stop is unsatisfactory, I visit two or three other places and then go to the diary to write down my notes and other observations.

I BREATHE LIKE A BUDDHA

Siddhartha Gautama, or the Buddha, is known worldwide for his ability to meditate for long periods.

Zen meditation and other related meditation practices are equally well known for teaching a deep breathing method that can relieve stress, banish fatigue, and increase concentration.

Deep, rhythmic breathing is the cornerstone of meditation and proper breathing, and I make my brain a world of good by giving it more oxygen to work with.

Breathing deeply and regularly means taking more oxygen and expelling more carbon dioxide and other unnecessary inert gases on the exhale.

Sometimes, I unknowingly fall into the bad habit of chest breathing, forcing air in and out by greatly expanding and contracting my chest. This is common for people like me who sit for long hours at a computer in a bad posture. The diaphragm and abdominal area become compressed, and the breath is not as deep. The result is tight chest muscles, low oxygen levels, and a feeling of fatigue that only we can truly understand.

I then consciously begin to breathe deeply, and here is what I do step by step.

1. I find a comfortable place to sit. Sometimes, I sit on a bed, on a chair or couch, on the living room floor, on the carpet, or

on a meditation or yoga mat. Anything is fine as long as I sit down and it is in a quiet place away from bright lights and loud sounds.

2. I sit up straight, arranging my spine like a stack of coins, keeping it in constant gentle movement and flow because it is just a stack of intervertebral discs. I don't need to be straight and still like a stick during this exercise, but I keep my back naturally erect because good posture also helps me breathe easier and be more present.

3. Now, I arrange my head, imagining it is connected to three giant balloons gently floating upwards. I let these balloons straighten my head and neck so my eyes look straight ahead. I then gently adjust my focus, hold it, or close my eyes.

4. When my back and head are straight, and I feel relaxed and ready to begin, I imagine my stomach as a giant balloon that fills with air when inhaled. As I inhale, I allow my abdominal region to expand horizontally while my thoracic region expands upwards. The two forms of expansion happen simultaneously; they are natural and keep me rested.

5. Deep breathing does not mean I must forcefully fill my lungs with air to burst. Deep breathing is conscious breathing that gets more air to clear my mind more easily. When I inhale, the air passes from my nostrils to my lungs, and vice versa when I exhale.

6. Now that I am gently engaged in deep breathing, I add meditation, which simply means that I pay attention to how the air moves in and out of me and that I pay attention to the fact that I am paying attention. I become aware of the flow of air and how it feels as I inhale and exhale; the sensation in my nostrils, the slight, gentle movement of air.

I practice this meditation technique for a few minutes: belly, nostrils, spine, awareness. Fifteen to twenty minutes is a good start. I don't think about what I am doing; I just do it and leave my mind peacefully and blissfully empty. I do this meditation exercise frequently, and my body remembers to breathe deeply throughout the day and night. It increases my ability to focus and ventilates my brain synapses.

Interested in Zen? Check out my books: Zen the Sense of Nonsense and Seeds of Enlightenment.

I MAKE A HABIT OF THINKING

If I can't compete with others in terms of strategy and implementation of my plans, the problem may be how I process information.

I can adopt a solid problem-solving mindset. In that case, all my worries and anxieties will surely vanish because I am more interested in finding real solutions to my situations and problems than worrying about them. This will benefit my brain, which operates on constructive and positive frequencies.

Critical thinking is the best mental strategy for dealing with what is happening to me, and it is the ultimate in problem-solving because I choose to be systematic when I deal with them.

For example, if I have a problem with my home gas consumption, I no longer worry about the issue and instead prefer to write it down on paper and think of ways to arrive at a solution. I don't have to be a mathematician or a scientist to find reasonable solutions. All I need is the desire to think critically and systematically, and the rest follows.

This is how I adopt a critical mindset.

1. When a problem bothers me, I don't ignore it or worry about it. I write it down on paper so I can address it directly.

2. After I write down the problem I want to address, I gather all the facts about it. I write them all down because these are the

tools I will later use to solve it. If I don't know much about the problem, I research or ask someone who knows the situation. I listen to what others say and memorize or record the new information. After gathering enough data, I move on to the next step.

3. Now it's time to step back and put all my worrying to rest. I then ask myself the following questions and write down the answers I come up with.

a. What would happen if I could solve this problem?

b. What would be the worst if I couldn't do anything about it anymore?

c. How can I get back on track after this problem?

Now that I have seen what could happen if this problem is not solved, I no longer have to worry because I have answered question c., which is my recovery and restoration plan. If my solutions don't work, I am already planning ahead because I want to recover from this problem.

4. I think of all the possible solutions to my problem. I list all the potential remedies I can think of, even the solutions that I don't think will work, because, at this point, I need all the possible formulas for success. So, I don't limit myself to a handful of solutions. If I can list a hundred, I will.

5. I choose a solution that will work and try it. If the problem is solved, I pat myself on the back and congratulate myself on my critical thinking, which has already paid off; if my first solution doesn't work, it simply means I need to go back to my list and select another solution. I continue until the problem is solved.

See my book, Imagine.

I LISTEN TO SELF-HYPNOSIS RECORDINGS

Hypnosis recordings are gaining a lot of traction these days because the audio engineering used by professional hypnotists has improved dramatically. In the past, they focused on integrating different elements into their personal hypnosis sessions with their patients. Today, I can download a library of great hypnosis recordings online.

All I need to do is listen to and benefit from them on my PC, laptop, MP3 player, or mobile phone. The latter is my favorite; I upload or download the recordings and listen to them whenever and wherever I want and whenever I have time.

The medical association has long supported the use of hypnosis in psychotherapy.

Hypnosis recordings usually use three elements: the script, an ambient music track, and reverberations that help deepen the hypnotic experience.

Hypnosis helps me restore my brain capacity in many ways, and the following are some of the situations in which I use it.

1. When I need to increase my level of concentration.

2. When I need to be more creative or free with my ideas and express myself through words, visual art, or music.

3. When I feel like I need to be more organized with my thoughts and words.

4. When I lack the confidence to express myself creatively in

front of others.

Hypnosis is the offspring of many disciplines, such as psychology and psychoanalysis, and is based on the fundamental principle that the human mind is strong enough to reprogram itself with the right tools.

Hypnosis is just a tool, and it is still up to me whether I want to accept the positive affirmations contained in the script of a hypnosis session. In fact, hypnosis does not work if I do not wish to take it or believe that it does not work.

Some circles of popular culture define hypnosis as a set of magic spells that take complete control of my mind; in reality, it is the opposite. Magic uses hypnosis, so no matter how powerful a hypnotic script is, I can still say no if I don't like what I feel and what it makes me think in the first place.

I prefer hypnosis to other forms of mental programming. For example, suppose I have to choose between hypnosis and subliminal messages. In that case, I like the former because subliminal seems still in the experimental stage with scattered studies on the subject, and I feel better knowing what I am letting penetrate my subconscious. Hypnosis, on the other hand, is already effectively used in hospitals around the world and is recognized not only by the medical profession but also by most of the alternative therapies approved by it today in our country.

I EXPLORE SPEED READING METHODS

Speed reading is a way of reading text using a system that allows me to get most ideas in individual paragraphs without reading the text typically, word by word.

Speed reading, like other self-taught systems, is highly recommended because it allows the brain to learn new skills and challenges the pre-existing system of gathering and processing information from the text being read.

I TALK TO MY SUBCONSCIOUS

My mind is divided into two main parts: the conscious or logical center and the subconscious or irrational level. As a child, my subconscious level of thought was often more powerful than the conscious logical center, so I was prone to flights of fancy.

Growing up, I was taught to suppress my subconscious because it is the seat of my deepest desires. These desires often clash with what society deems acceptable and correct. Still, the subconscious seat of the mind is also the seat of my natural creativity and curiosity, which, if I continue to consciously suppress and disconnect, will eventually become less functional and eventually shut down.

A beautiful strategy for reconnecting with my subconscious, so simple it seems obvious, is to talk to it. It may seem bizarre, but I really gain a tremendous amount of information and wisdom from it. I talk to my subconscious by giving it a voice, and sometimes I give it a shape or a face; I build a character and make it my friend, my subconscious companion.

I talk to the character in my mind. It is clear that I am talking to myself, but with a side of me that is relatively unknown, and I apply an extra effort to understand its meanings, language, symbols, and what my subconscious mind wants to tell me. We talk before going to sleep so that the night brings counsel; we talk when we wake up when the mind is fresh and rested; we talk when necessary so that I use the immense amount of information and knowledge in my subconscious.

I SOLVE PUZZLES REGULARLY

I used to dislike puzzles. They are designed to confuse me, and it sometimes takes a long time before I can fully solve them. But regardless of what I may have thought about these games, solving puzzles is still a fantastic way to reset my brain. When I solve crosswords, Sudoku, and countless other puzzles, I challenge my brain in ways it has never been challenged before, thus allowing it to use new cognitive resources to arrive at the correct answer. The frustration I feel when solving puzzles is my mind searching for answers. I am frustrated because, on the surface, I don't get the answers right away, but deep down, my mind is still working full force and tirelessly to solve the puzzle itself. The best time to solve puzzles is during downtime, which is a lousy way of saying it: in between situations. Downtime is free time during the day and can last minutes or hours, depending on the situation. For example, if I wait 20 minutes for the bus, I start a Sudoku game and solve it. My phone is full of great games downloaded for free from the Internet. I choose the exciting ones and play them almost whenever I am free.

Of course, I get the most significant brain benefits when I solve puzzles for extended periods; practice sharpens my wits and strengthens my brain. Sometimes, I can play for just 5 minutes a day; this is also fine; it keeps me on the right track, and the benefits add up over time. It is true.

I AM MORE AWARE OF WHO I AM

How well do I know myself, apart from the usual things like what I like to eat, what clothes I consider fashionable, what I have studied, and so on?

If I think this is an unimportant factor in restoring my brain's capacity, I am wrong because it is essential. A lack of self-awareness increases the risk of letting unhelpful beliefs control my thinking.

When I have a lot of emotional baggage and false beliefs, my mind tends to prioritize these well-established beliefs, even when they don't contribute to my problem-solving process. Improving my self-awareness literally increases my brain's ability to repair itself because, from now on, I am not hindered by emotional baggage and underlying false beliefs.

See my book, The Secret of Meditation.

SELF-MOTIVATION IS ESSENTIAL

If I want to learn something new or solve a complicated problem, I have to tell and convince myself that I can do so that my brain responds accordingly. I use my imagination to my advantage.

My brain cannot distinguish between what is in my imagination and what is happening and is quite capable of accepting what I imagine as reality. So, if I motivate myself by imagining that I can solve a problem, I can do it.

The easiest way to motivate my mind is to create positive affirmations. These are simply beliefs that I repeat to myself when I need them.

Here are some examples of positive affirmations that I use.

I am a bestselling author.

I lose up to 70 kg in a few months.

I lower my blood pressure naturally.

I reduce my cholesterol through a proper diet.

I am confident in any social situation.

I can solve math problems quickly.

I sell anything to anyone.

I am the best employee in this company.

I am the best at what I do.

I solve problems like a pro.

I unleash my inner leader.

Positive affirmations focus on what I want to accomplish in the present and future. They keep me grounded and motivated because my positive affirmations remain the same even if I struggle with what I do.

STRESS ULTIMATELY LOWERS MY BRAIN CAPACITY

Stress is neither a disease nor something I can give to others like a cold virus. Stress is a natural physiological response in the body, and I get stressed when I feel in danger. Thousands of years ago, stress as a physiological response was beneficial because my ancestors lived in hostile environments.

Stress is a physiological response that is part of the survival instinct package that life has given us. It usually kicks in and out when I can escape danger or deal with what is threatening me.

For example, if a tiger threatens me and my family unit, stress comes into play because I must be more aggressive than the aggressor or get away from the danger as quickly as possible. When the tiger is gone, there is no stress either, and the body, mind, and spirit return to normal as the physiological response to danger dissipates.

As a social human, I have evolved by leaps and bounds in some aspects of my life, but I have always remained the same in others. One of my great acts of success is to continue to recreate an environment that allows me to get into stress, even if the external triggering need is missing. The facts and problems of life are complex and intersect, and I tend to feel stressed, even if the source of stress is miles away, such as at work or years away, such as when I was a child or as I will be in old age.

There is a big difference between the stress of real danger and the stress of these days, and I can no longer find the switch to turn it off. In fact, I am often stressed even when I sleep. Sometimes, I am so tired of dealing with and managing stress hormones and all the other changes that happen to me when I am in a stressed state that my body eventually gets sick. Stress also kills my mental acuity and concentration because my body, mind, emotions, and spirit are all preoccupied with sustaining the physiological stress response to the threat or danger, real or imagined.

Prolonged stress over the years can actually damage my brain, and I need to be aware of that, especially when I let myself get so stressed that I feel like I am going to explode or collapse from the mounting pressure.

I need to prioritize stress management at work, school, and home. Stress is the number one secret killer, and excessive stress is known to contribute to degenerative severe conditions like high blood pressure and other cardiovascular diseases.

But I am ready to deal with it, and here is how I will do it.

1. If I can, I take control of the current situation. I may have little power to solve situations I don't like, but there is always room for personal action. If I am willing to take action and speak up, there is usually something I can contribute to a stressful situation. For example, I am constantly stressed at home because I find that everything is messed up instead of overreacting and yelling at everyone. In that case, I simply hold a family meeting to air my complaints with whoever is responsible for the confusion and my subsequent stress. After airing my complaints, I use my critical mind to draft possible solutions to my problem. Usually, the tension dissipates when everyone finally puts their issues on the table, and a solution is in the works. This approach suits me better than pretending that nothing is wrong or going crazy every single day; in both cases, I am, in fact, at a loss because I am still stressed and the problem has not been resolved.

2. I set practical, achievable goals. Many contemporary experts preach that setting goals is essential to achieve anything in this life. Some are even so bold as to say that the more goals I have, the more fulfilled I will be. Achieving goals is undoubtedly an excellent way to manifest my dreams, but too many goals at once also cause me a lot of stress. I live in an age of instant gratification that places a high value on things that bring immediate benefits. I forget that good things take time to manifest and that nothing is ever genuinely given in an instant.

Sometimes, I get the insatiable itch to indulge in more good things in the short term. This is my leading cause of burnout and stress, which has deleterious effects on my brain and health. This is precisely why I create fewer goals for myself. I stick to the goals that will bring me accumulated rewards and discard the rest for now. Having fewer goals means I cannot work on multiple goals simultaneously.

3. I learned to walk away from things that cause me stress. Stress itself is not something that just mingles with the air and infects everyone; stress is always caused by something. I may not be able to pinpoint the cause right now, but these causative factors are all around me and within me. As I have already seen, the trick is to first identify what is causing me stress at home or work and disconnect from that source regularly to restore myself.

Disconnecting from stressors is not difficult at all. For example, if my children are causing me pain with all the brutality they commit, I disconnect from the stressful situation by taking a short walk outside the house. I walk for five or ten minutes and then return to solve the problem. I am still amazed at how much disconnecting from stress helps me manage it; my mind is more precise, all the harsh and negative emotions inside me dissipate along with the stress, and my brain relaxes and smiles.

4. I do not pretend to be Superman. I admit it: I can't be a perfect husband, employee, parent, gamer, child, or entrepreneur all the time. Sometimes, my mental and physical energy isn't enough to accomplish all that. If I feel like I'm

about to be a disaster at everything I do, I stop. That's right; I stop because I need to reevaluate what's truly important on my long to-do list.

If I constantly feel like I need to be in three places at once, there's something seriously wrong with how I've structured my life. I then review what needs to be prioritized and decide what to let go of. For example, it's not the end of the world if I can't attend a community fundraising because I have to take care of the kids or the dog.

It's a matter of prioritizing what I can do, and I create different priorities. Level one is the things I need to do now because there will be consequences if I don't get them done; level two is the things I need to get done soon but can wait a few days or weeks; and level three is the things I need to get done soon but can wait a few more days or weeks. And finally, the third tier is what I can deal with now, but it doesn't have far-reaching consequences if I leave it out indefinitely.

See my book, The Art of Worrying.

I AM HUNGRY FOR NEW INFORMATION

I often ignore things happening around me because I have too much going on right now to be curious. If I want a solid brain reset, asking questions is one of the easiest ways to stimulate my brain regularly. The questions don't have to be groundbreaking or complicated; they just have to be frequent so that my brain is stimulated often.

For example, if I see a guy giving a girl a bouquet of flowers and the girl receiving the flowers can't make eye contact or even speak, and the guy also doesn't respond to the fact that the woman doesn't seem to be interested in what just happened, what kind of questions might come to mind when I see a situation like that? I mustn't get caught up in the problem I'm observing; I'm simply stimulating my mind by asking myself many questions.

If I can answer them, that's fine. It means that my brain is ready for further input and is rapidly recalling facts and understandings from my memory to answer my questions. This is a little exercise I also practice when I watch television, whether it's the news or movies; there are always twists and turns in the current story or the plot that I keep guessing until the end of the program.

I PRIORITIZE MY BRAIN RESTORATION

Restoring my brain capacity is not an overnight event, and even if I play solitaire all night, it builds up little by little. It is an ongoing process, much like bodybuilding, that requires regular work on the brain's muscles to achieve the desired results, equivalent to the amount of effort I put into restoring my brain capacity.

This brings me to a fundamental point in all my work, which I summarize with this phrase: I need to have a plan of action to ensure that I always remember that I am actually trying to restore my brain capacity. I choose a few sustainable and actionable strategies if I can't commit to significant lifestyle changes.

For example, if I can't commit to buying natural brain supplements and organic food, I at least get enough rest every day and try to avoid fatty and sugary foods. If I can't learn to play a new musical instrument due to time constraints, I choose an equally valid strategy, such as reading more books in my spare time or solving more puzzles to stimulate my mind and brain.

When I make plans like this, I write down my thoughts in my journal so I can review and possibly adjust my plan of action. I can always change my strategies if some need to be fixed.

See my book, The Art of Change.

A CHANGE OF SCENARIO

As a human, I am always looking for stability and security, yet I also paradoxically need to be in different environments to avoid mental stagnation.

Being in one place my whole life really fossilizes my mental ability. My brain stagnates and becomes unmotivated, and I feel the contracted effect of being stuck in one environment for long months or years.

As a human, I am a social being and a curious natural traveler. I am happiest when I can visit other places to learn more about the world and, in the process, myself.

Traveling is not a luxury; it is a need. When I travel, I am often happier, more contented, and more intelligent because I have seen the world and have more perspectives and opinions to share with others.

I need to plan this year's travel itinerary when I want a fantastic learning experience that will restore my brain power. By travel, I don't mean spending big bucks visiting faraway countries. Wherever I live, my country offers a wide variety of places to visit that are enough for an average traveler.

Here are some guiding questions I ask myself to help me determine the perfect places to visit this year.

1. What places have I dreamed of visiting since I was young? Are these places realistic to see this year? If so, which are these

places, and when do I plan to visit them?

2. What historical monuments in my country do I want to see? Is there any personal reason why I want to see these historical places?

3. What interests me the most? I am interested in music. Is there a particular city I would like to visit because of its history and local culture?

4. If I could choose only one country to visit for fun and relaxation, which would it be?

Now, I chose Asia.

I FEED MY BRAIN

In this part of the book, I focus on feeding my brain by selecting healthy, specific, and unique foods. My brain needs proper nutrition, and the saying reminds me that the brain receives what I give to the body in general; therefore, if my diet consists mainly of high-calorie junk food, devoid of essential nutrients, full of sugary drinks and dairy products, I do not expect or demand that my brain will be as brilliant as it was years ago.

My brain is a massive bundle of specialized cells that retain, recall, and defragment information and ensure that I do not fall when I walk. It is the very center of my thought processes and emotions. If I do not give it proper nutrition or at least some adequate nutrition, I cannot expect it to be as sharp and creative as ever.

I use several brain foods to restore it to its former health. Although these foods were not chosen because they can physically heal the brain, they are known to improve thought processes and various brain functions. Of course, I prefer the ones that best suit my lifestyle and personal tastes and integrate them into my daily diet. I also realize that no existing food can restore my brain power in a week; the natural approach requires patience and consistency, and therefore, I must integrate it into my lifestyle to get long-term benefits. Here are the foods I use.

COCOA

The much-loved chocolate bar is partly derived from the cocoa bean. However, I do not eat large amounts of chocolate just to get the cocoa content.

Many cocoa products are less processed than chocolate bars, such as cocoa drinks made from cocoa pressed into hard bars, fine powder, and other similar food products.

I am aware that cocoa is not as sweet and buttery as the chocolate I am familiar with and that it is actually bitter, but I am not looking for the taste, but the benefits for my brain.

Current research suggests that cocoa—not processed chocolate products—is a complete health agent that protects my cognitive function, skin, and heart.

Cocoa is also rich in antioxidants, which are necessary for optimal health. The easiest way to benefit from this age-old health food is to mix cocoa powder with any existing beverage, such as coffee.

It doesn't matter if it tastes bitter; if I don't like bitter, I think about how cocoa helps my thinking process in the long run.

MATCHA (GREEN TEA POWDER)

I've been drinking tea for a while now, and that's good because all forms of tea are packed with antioxidants that help prevent free radicals from taking over healthy tissue in my body.

Tea is a popular health drink that has been shown to prevent certain diseases and prolong life. In fact, a study in Japan a few years ago showed that people who drank tea 4-5 times a day lived much longer than those who didn't.

I'm taking it up a notch. If I want to restore my brainpower, I will invest in something more potent than commercial tea bags.

I need matcha, which is really just the ground tea plant. While most other teas are brewed by steeping the tea leaves in boiling or near-boiling water and removing them after several minutes, with matcha, I stir and dissolve it and drink it with the water.

Matcha has long been used in Buddhist ceremonies, and monks routinely drink it to maintain health and stay alert during long meditations. A key matcha component is L-theanine, which I am looking for.

Because of the tea they drink, monks who drink matcha can focus on their meditation practices for more than 10 hours at a time. Putting that kind of concentrated power into my work increases my average productivity by leaps and bounds.

Matcha also contains epigallocatechin gallate, which is long heralded as a powerful anti-aging compound that protects against radiation. Combining it with a healthy lifestyle benefits my brain from this small change.

ACAI BERRY

Many products on the market promise the world, but in most cases, they prove to be less effective than expected. One exception is the acai berry, which is used by so many different companies that it can make you nervous just hearing the name. But it is not the berry's fault that I take advantage of its health benefits.

The acai berry is on my list of foods to restore my brain's capabilities for the following reasons.

1. It contains the highest level of natural antioxidants compared to other commercially available berries.

2. It contains incredibly high protein levels, which is unusual for a fruit.

3. Due to its nutritional profile, it is considered a superfood.

To get all the benefits of the acai berry, I eat it fresh or frozen, but if it is not available in those forms, I settle for what I find on the market. I also avoid products that claim to have a percentage of acai berry because I don't need to process it when I can have it naturally.

BLUEBERRIES

If I can't get acai berries, I switch to a more well-known fruit equally helpful in healing the brain: the blueberry.

Not the one in desserts, which, when I overeat, causes discomfort to my body by introducing high levels of sugar and dietary fat.

I eat blueberries fresh, with little or no additives. A cup of blueberries daily is the supreme natural multivitamin that nature has given me.

COFFEE BEANS

Coffee beans are as excellent as cocoa beans because real coffee—without the sugar, cream, and everything else I add to the final blend—is a superfood because of its high amount of nutrients. Recent studies show that drinking coffee is not only good for your body overall but also for your brain.

In fact, research shows that regular coffee consumption helps prevent age-related degenerative conditions that affect not only your mental stability but also the structure of your brain itself.

Coffee is a healthy food primarily because it provides a steady stream of antioxidants and contains caffeine, naturally stimulating your body and brain. To get the benefits of coffee without the unhealthy risks of everything I add, I buy high-quality coffee beans, grind them, and make my coffee at home.

I drink it without cream, artificial sweeteners, or copious amounts of milk and sugar, and I'm well on my way to a healthier mind. I give my brain something that prevents disease and helps directly stimulate it.

WHOLE GRAIN PRODUCTS

I love bread and pasta but have switched to whole-grain products for the best health benefits while enjoying my macaroni or spaghetti at home. Anything whole grain is a good choice for me and nourishes me deeply.

This particular evaluation is because whole grain foods contain a lot of B vitamins and folate.

These vitamins are necessary for normal body functions, and recent studies show that increasing your intake of foods rich in these essential nutrients improves memory recall compared to those who do not eat diets rich in B vitamins and folate.

TOMATOES

I love tomatoes. These versatile fruits are used in so many dishes that I don't notice them anymore, except when they are missing. Tomatoes are rich in lycopene, a powerful antioxidant shown to protect the brain and help prevent degenerative conditions like dementia.

In addition to lycopene, a single tomato contains the following nutrients.

Vitamin C, Vitamin K, Vitamin A, Potassium, Iron, Tryptophan, Vitamin E, Copper, Fiber, Manganese, Niacin.

That's actually only half of the good stuff in a tomato. It's no wonder it's hailed as one of the best superfoods in the world, providing me with tons of benefitsi.

BLACKCURRANT

I love blackcurrants and eat them regularly, and I'm happy to know that I've actually done my brain a lot of good. Blackcurrants are a great source of ascorbic acid, or vitamin C.

Vitamin C protects my lungs and immune system from damage from external agents and helps my brain become more agile when processing memories and sensory input. And while you can't take vitamin C specifically to treat severe brain conditions, it is recommended as a vitamin that can restore brain function over time.

CHIA SEEDS

Looking for a vegetarian source of omega-3 fatty acids, I came across chia seeds. These seeds are concentrated sources of omega-3, which helps my heart be healthier, and my brain becomes more efficient.

I eat chia seeds as they are in salads. When I make it, I put them in whole wheat bread and integrate them everywhere in my daily diet.

The same goes for flax seeds.

NATURAL RECOVERY SUPPLEMENTS

The fruits, vegetables, and foods I consume often come from faraway places; they are intensively grown, harvested prematurely, ripened in refrigerators during transport, and generally contain fewer nutrients than they did decades ago. For these reasons, I periodically take multivitamins and multimineral supplements to provide for the daily needs of my body, mind, and spirit. In this regard, I am free to choose the ones that I like the most, and the information is available almost everywhere, on the Internet, at the supermarket, and in the pharmacy; but regarding the restoration of my brain capacity, two particular plants interest me quite a bit, and they are Gingko Biloba and St. John's Wort.

Ginkgo Biloba – which is also at risk of extinction, and therefore, if I use it, I help save the species – has long been revered as one of the medicinal wonders because of all the conditions that tradition indicates it can benefit. Whether ginkgo biloba, as it is said, cures everything remains to be seen, but for thousands of years, the infusion of this root has been drunk to improve concentration and the thought process.

I am not allergic to it, so I searched for and found the one that works for me among the many supplements. Recent studies have shown that ginkgo biloba increases the blood supply to the brain by increasing blood flow. It is a widely cultivated plant and, for this reason, relatively cheap compared to other supplements. The daily intake is contained in one or two tablets or capsules.

More blood to the brain means more oxygen, and oxygen is food for the brain, which never has enough because it constantly sends chemical and electrical signals to every body part to keep everything functioning normally.

The other supplement is St. John's Wort (Hypericum). This particular supplement has been around for a few decades, and while it doesn't directly help restore my brain energy, it is used to treat depression and, therefore, helps my brain stay happy, which is essential for me if I want to think and work well.

Research proves that taking St. John's Wort has a temporary mood-altering effect. This simply means that if I'm feeling a little tense or down, for example, from increasing pressure at work, St. John's Wort herbal tea helps me get back on track.

Of course, before taking new supplements, I always ask my GP for advice, who, following my tests, is happy to advise me on products and dosages. In fact, some supplements, even if they are herbal or plant-derived, are powerful, and it is always good to know if they are compatible with other supplements or medications.

IN SUMMARY

Why Do I Pay Attention To My Brain?

My human brain is an incredible processing machine, and the number of connections within it exceeds the connections of any supercomputer today. I am only just beginning to understand how this powerful organ of mine works.

My brain is responsible for the normal functioning of my entire human body. It is often the last organ to fail in situations of injury and extreme stress and is one of the most resilient organs. Even during times of severe physical trauma, my human brain fights desperately to ensure the survival of my entire body.

As an average human, I only use a small percentage of my total brain capacity, meaning a vast cognitive resource inside my skull is waiting to be unleashed. Unlocking the true potential of my human mind is simple, and, in fact, I am already starting to do so.

Restoring my brain's capabilities is actually an ongoing process. There is no one way to do it; all strategies are built differently according to how I respond to them in different life cycles.

Another exceptional truth I am happy to know is that when I regularly challenge and stimulate my human brain, it finds reasons to grow and expand. Neural connections increase, and I become more mentally sharp and capable, no matter how old or young I am. If I really want this to happen, I will work to make it happen with the right strategies to restore my brain capacity.

Healthy Eating Restores My Brain Capacity

The first step to permanently restoring my brain capacity is to change my diet to eat healthier and more nutritious foods and less junk food. By junk food, I mean primarily fatty and sugary products. Most processed foods are also low in essential nutrients and macronutrients like protein, so I also pay attention to those. Brain capacity begins not in the brain itself but in the stomach. My body and brain are only as healthy as the food I eat.

I Drink Matcha To Restore My Mind

Of all the commercial beverages today, few come close to matcha's health benefits. Matcha is just green tea, but it is not consumed like other forms of commercial tea.

I usually use tea in permeable paper tea bags. There is nothing wrong with commercial tea bags, but if I want to get a considerable boost of antioxidants every time I drink tea, I need to find a good matcha shop and start stocking my kitchen cabinets with them.

Matcha is green tea ground into an excellent powder. Unlike regular tea, the green tea plants used to make matcha are grown in the shade, away from sunlight.

These shade-grown plants produce more chlorophyll and amino acids than other tea plants that bask in the sun. The pickers then choose only the most perfect leaves for final production.

Of course, the most reliable matcha sources are in countries like Japan, so I am careful when purchasing matcha from websites and do my research before they ship it to my home.

Matcha is known to increase mental acuity and concentration when consumed regularly. In fact, monks who are engaged in long religious rituals drink matcha to stay alert and focused, and it has been done for hundreds, if not thousands, of years, so matcha has a long history of effectiveness. If my doctor advises me against drinking too much coffee, matcha is my good alternative.

I Organize My Scattered Ideas With Mind Maps

One of the biggest problems I face when planning is having trouble putting my ideas together. Simply listing my ideas doesn't solve this. The tool that helps me most in this situation is a mind map.

A mind map is an organized blueprint of ideas that allows me to create expansive diagrams with pen and paper. The idea behind a mind map is that I can plan something if I can make the right connections between the multitudes of ideas in my head.

I don't need to buy specialized software to achieve this. All I need is a large sheet of paper, preferably a sketchbook, pen, pencil, or marker. I stick firmly to manually creating my mind maps to get a broad range of feelings and an overview before moving on to more restrictive and limited mind mapping software, like those on my phone.

A mind map consists of headings, subheadings, and associated ideas. That's it. With these three main elements, I organize my ideas about anything.

I plan my travel itinerary or build that dream boat I've always wanted. No matter how difficult or complex the problem is, with a mind map, all my ideas are organized into clusters and groups of data, neatly arranged for easy reference and editing.

The Benefits of Keeping a Journal

Sometimes, my job causes me fatigue and stress, but while I can't escape the reality that I have to work for a decent living, I can still ensure that my mind and body remain healthy even when there are increasing pressures at work.

When I feel burned out from work and clearly notice that my mind has also suffered from endless days of hard work, I start writing in my journal, which works wonders. I keep the journal with me and simply fill the pages with words.

Journaling is one of the longest-used therapies for stress and anxiety management, and now experts are seeing that it also restores brain power. Here are some of the main benefits of journaling.

1. It helps me improve my cognitive function.

2. Journaling boosts my immune system, which helps reduce my chances of getting sick from common ailments like the flu.

3. Regular journaling helps me reduce asthma attacks, arthritis pain, hysteria, etc.

4. Journaling helps me combat the impact of stress on my body and mind.

I am starting a journal today; I just need a lovely journal. Countless shops and stationery stores sell superb journals at desirable prices. I browse the Internet and find a journal there that I really like, and in this way, I enjoy writing in it more and more.

I Don't Forget Naps

Some people tell me they don't need much sleep and feel fine after 4 or 5 hours. Not only is this bad for my body, it seems that my chances of a heart attack or stroke increase when I only get 5 hours of sleep a night, but it's also bad for my human mind.

No matter how smart or clever I am, my mental acuity takes a hit if I don't give my body enough rest each night. My human brain can only compensate for so much tiredness, after which it slowly gives up and ceases to be efficient.

I don't worry if I haven't slept well in the past few years; there's always a chance to catch up. All I do is adjust my sleep patterns so that I start going to bed earlier; 10 pm/11pm is ideal for me, and I start waking up earlier; 6 am/7am is a great time to wake up when I've gone to bed early at night.

If I can't change my sleep habits right now, the least I can do to maintain my mental acuity is to nap daily. I take really great mid-day naps.

I can squeeze in a quarter of an hour of nap time in the middle of the day, and it's enough to give my body and mind some much-needed rest. I can nap for 30 minutes or more, providing immediate benefits in increased focus and faster information processing.

I Meditate For A Restored Mind

Meditation is one of the few alternative health practices that actually gives me immediate results when I practice it. Meditation is an ancient art that combines progressive relaxation, rhythmic breathing, and strategic postures.

Zen meditation is one of the most popular forms of meditation worldwide, and I join thousands of practitioners worldwide. Meditation is not tied to any religious beliefs, so I don't worry if it crosses my mind that this practice is occult. Research has shown that meditation helps me focus better on my tasks because it naturally clears mental fog.

It's actually easy to start meditating. Here's how I meditate at home.

1. I find a comfortable chair to sit in and straighten my back so I don't slump or hunch forward.

2. I focus on a point on the wall before me to keep my head up and my neck straight.

3. I breathe exclusively through the nostrils because the breath is fuller if I practice it through the nostrils.

4. When I inhale, I allow my abdominal region to expand well, followed by the thoracic region. I imagine my abdominal region swelling from the inside, and I want it to extend well to let in the oxygen that gives me life.

5. I pay close attention to the movement of the air as it passes through the nose and concentrate on the movement itself during inhalation and exhalation. That is all I do. I practice this exercise every day, 5 to 8 minutes per session, extending it to an hour when I have the time and desire to be quiet.

A Fit Body Produces a Fit Mind

A decade ago, I thought that my body was clearly separate from my mind and that this was a good thing since my mind had some form of independence from my human body. I believed this until medical science started to disprove this theory.

Current studies show that the connection between the mind and the body is so strong that if something terrible happens to the body, the mind also suffers. Conversely, my brain benefits immensely if I do something good for my body.

This led me to realize that I need exercise to enhance my human mind. I incorporate regular exercise into my daily routine to keep my body and mind fit and strong. Medical science now recommends exercise for many conditions because it just works. Exercise not only burns off excess calories, but it also helps keep my brain stimulated and healthy.

The mind-body connection is real, so I pay attention to this approach. I want my brain to be in order, and I achieve this by first strengthening my body. The brain then receives the same benefits as the rest of the organs in my body.

I don't lift barbells and other heavyweights to get a good workout; I dance and do mixed martial arts. I ensure that my chosen activity is the cornerstone of my new physical fitness regimen. I exercise regularly, 3-5 times a week.

Video Games Restore My Brain Power

If I thought in my thirties or forties that games of any kind no longer had a place in my life simply because I was too old for such things, I was wrong. If I avoid all types of games, I miss an excellent opportunity to sharpen my mind and improve my cognitive abilities.

That's right. Games actually help me restore my brain power. There are no hard and fast rules regarding the types of games I play. If I like first or third-person shooters, then by all means, I play war games. If I prefer challenging puzzle games, that's a good choice, too. The important thing is that I allow my mind to explore a completely different type of stimulation. When my human brain is challenged with new situations and problems, it creates more neural networks to adapt to new situations more easily. My brain wants to be challenged and enjoys these mental challenges. I don't mind being stumped when solving puzzles and the like. The essential result when I play games is allowing my mind to solve different problems, which is the equivalent of a brain workout. Games keep my brain stimulated and alert, ready for the next challenge.

Socializing Is Important For My Mental Health Too

One of the best ways to restore my brain power is to socialize with other people more regularly, not by chatting on the phone or online but by meeting them in real life and hanging out with the people I want to be with.

Isolating myself from others harms my human mind because I am, by nature, a social being. My human mind needs constant social interaction.

Current studies confirm this, and, in fact, recent research shows that when I socialize regularly, I am less at risk of many degenerative health conditions, such as dementia, in my later years.

This is because regular social interactions are a natural source of sensory stimulation. My brain feeds off my experiences interacting with others and remains robust and efficient when I ensure that stimulation is provided regularly.

I don't have to spend much money to reach out to the people who matter to me. A simple get-together at home is good enough for my brain. I don't spend much money just because I want to socialize more.

Of course, since I can afford it, I do so by inviting and arranging, but for the most part, my focus is solely on interacting with friends, colleagues, family, and new acquaintances.

APPENDIX 1

Restoring My Brain Capacity Now

Restoring my brain capacity requires ongoing effort over time. There are no overnight quick fixes, but there are many strategies I can employ to ensure my brain is adequately stimulated by suitable activities. I will follow these great strategies and start restoring my brain capacity now.

I challenge one or more of my senses. Too often, I rely on just one or two senses, usually hearing and sight. However, when I intentionally block my primary senses, my brain works harder to compensate for my missing senses. Blocking one or more senses is good brain exercise. I practice this simple brain reset technique when I do simple activities like eating or even when I'm folding origami.

Not when driving or using machines, but otherwise, I can blindfold myself or plug my ears with earplugs without any problems. During the exercise, I immersed myself in the experience of using my other senses to make sense of what was happening. The longer I immerse myself in the exercise, the better the results.

I discover new uses for ordinary objects. This tremendous mental exercise brings me many creative benefits and costs me nothing. It identifies an everyday object I want to focus on, such as a chair, table, clock, keys, plastic case, phone, shadows, plastic figurines, or lighter.

Once I've chosen a mundane object, I take a piece of paper and a pencil and write down other alternative uses.

I don't write down things I already know, such as using the chair to sit on. I think of crazy and bizarre uses for my chosen everyday object. If I find 10 uses, I try to write down 10 more. I write until my creativity is completely drained and then move on to the following everyday object.

I embark on a sensory adventure. I live visually centered and trust my eyes more than all my other senses, which leads to long-term mental stagnation and reduced acuity. I need to use all my senses to keep my mind sharp, and I do this in many ways.

For example, I visit a bakery to taste cookies and breads that I would never have thought of buying for myself. I challenge my sense of smell by blindfolding myself and having a friend bring me things to smell that I have to identify by nose alone.

I want to expand my other senses to challenge my brain further and give me the correct answer. I quickly embark on a sensory adventure anywhere, at home or on the go. I practice this exercise once or more a week and am well on my way to restoring my brain power.

APPENDIX 2

How I Restore My Mental Abilities

As an adult, I often dream of being mentally sharp and agile again. Unfortunately, my poor lifestyle choices and even my worst thinking habits cause my mental decline to the point where I feel like I can no longer organize my thoughts well or express myself creatively. It doesn't have to be this way because I use simple daily strategies to improve my brain power. Here are some of the techniques I use to restore my mental abilities.

I change my diet. If I want a healthy mind, I first need a healthy body, and the easiest way to achieve that is to improve and change my diet. When I eat healthy foods daily, my mind is sharp enough; I only need to perform a few mental exercises to restore it a little more. When I do not eat well, I immediately change my diet as soon as possible by eliminating anything processed and sticking to healthy, home-cooked meals. The more I cook at home, the more control I have over what I put into my body. If I eat out, I am limited by the menu at the restaurant or cafe. When shopping, I also choose a rainbow of fruits and vegetables and organic foods; I eat nuts, dried fruit, and yogurt, all good for my brain.

I get adequate sleep every night. Nothing can bog down my brain more than physical exhaustion. My body needs sufficient rest to keep my mind strong and agile. In addition, my mind needs rest, too. I typically need 7 to 8 hours of sleep every night as an adult. I go to bed relatively early and wake up early. This is my best practice. I produce more results in the morning, so I wake up early daily. If I sleep better, my brainpower definitely improves in a short period.

I listen to music. If I always feel tired and anxious due to increasing pressure at work, the best way to deal with stress is to listen to music. If I can handle stress well, my mind will stay healthy, strong, and creative. If I let the pressures at work touch and penetrate me, my mind gets bogged down, and I always feel tired and weak. I choose a genre of music that relaxes me and alternate emotional songs with softer ones. Listening to music should be therapeutic and not overly stimulating. I listen to music before bed so I can fall asleep more easily. Music calms my tired mind and helps me rest all night.

APPENDIX 3

Restoring My Brain Power

When I want to restore my brain power, I know that I can't do it overnight and need to work on it regularly to get quick results. Restoring my brain power is like strengthening my muscles; I need to train my brain frequently if I want it to get bigger and stronger.

Here are some strategies I use to get started on the right foot.

I play games and do quizzes. Current research shows that games effectively stimulate and challenge my human mind. In addition to video games and more conventional games like chess, I solve puzzles like crosswords, Sudoku, and riddles. The more challenging the game, the harder my brain works to find the right solutions, and when the brain is challenged, it creates new neural connections to adapt to the increased need to process complicated information. Countless game programs on the market offer excellent, challenging solutions. Naturally, I choose the ones that are the most enjoyable for me.

I play at being ambidextrous. I usually work with just my dominant hand, mainly for comfort. However, it is possible to become ambidextrous and use both of my hands to draw, write, brush my teeth, eat, operate my phone, remote control, mouse, and so on. I teach myself to become ambidextrous. It's amazing how much hard work my brain puts into teaching my other hand the tasks that have been relegated to my dominant hand. Even if I fail immediately, which is normal, I constantly learn something new.

I enjoy and appreciate my ambiguities. Too often, I stick to my comfort zone regarding food, clothing, thoughts, and even the things I pay attention to. I leave my comfort zone and look for things outside my old pattern. I read more fiction and nonfiction to broaden my creative horizons, and I embrace the weird, always trying to learn from new experiences.

I value my mind maps. Mind mapping is beneficial for me when I have trouble organizing my thoughts and ideas. Mind maps are just diagrams that I use to connect my multitude of ideas to each other. It's a way to express myself and simultaneously organize what's going through my head. The best thing about mind maps is that I can easily edit them whenever a group of ideas isn't working for me. I just delete those groups or clusters to remove them. With my mind maps, I connect small groups of ideas to other headings and subsections of my thinking. Ultimately, I connect ten or twenty ideas and follow what I originally planned. For example, if I'm planning to build a new boat, I use a mind map to make sure I can cope with all the parts of the ship, with all the materials and tools that go with it.

APPENDIX 4

Restoring My Mental Capacity

As I age, my mind tends to become slower and less creative, but it doesn't have to be that way. I can be sharper than ever in my fifties if I want to. I just have to put in the extra effort to achieve that. I get the desired results if I start my practices early to restore my mental capacity. Here are some tremendous mental restoration strategies I use to get started.

I practice critical thinking. Too often, I rely on my pre-established answers for different situations. If a problem arises, I refer to standard solutions and then move on. But this way, they live my life without using my critical faculties. In the long run, my creativity and logical thinking suffer because they were never fully utilized. But that's already in the past, and right now, I'm learning to adopt a critical mindset. Here's how.

1. I always ask questions. When I ask questions, I reshape reality and gain the potential and alternatives within a given situation. I accept other people's beliefs and solutions if I don't ask questions frequently. This is convenient sometimes, but it doesn't help me restore my mental energy because I restore a passive acceptance of information instead.

2. I systematically solve problems. Whenever I face a problem, the best thing I can do is first list everything I know

about the issue, then I list all the possible solutions. If my current solution doesn't work, I move on and try other solutions from my list.

3. I don't immediately believe what I see or hear. Often, things aren't really what they seem. I find it wrong to trust what I see because my situations are usually manipulated just to get my approval. So, before I accept something as the truth, I am curious and try to grasp the truth behind what appears before me.

I'm drawing more frequently. Drawing is just one of my fun ways to express myself. I don't need to be good at drawing because this is also an exercise to restore my brain capacity. I bought a nice big sketch pad to draw more on a page. I draw when I feel happy, sad, angry, or like drawing. I use drawing as a vehicle to express my thoughts and emotions, and my brain works hard to express itself through lines and shapes.

I think positively. If I think negatively most of the time, I will attract negative things into my life. This is the core of the law of attraction. I have to think positively if I want to attract positive things into my life, and I have to think positively if I want my mind to come up with great solutions to my problems because if I keep thinking that I can't solve something, eventually my brain agrees with that side of me.

APPENDIX 5

Restoring My Brain

I have been wondering how to restore my brain power without spending much money on seminars and personal tutoring, and I can do it now. Everything I need to regain my ability to process information and recall facts is already at my fingertips. I just need to know the strategies that help me achieve my goals. Below are some excellent ones that help me achieve my brain restoration goals.

I am more creative and express myself in different ways. My human brain has two main divisions representing two distinct thinking centers: the creative and the logical.

I often use the logical center of my brain for problem-solving, planning events, rationalizing, judging, etc., while I use the creative center mainly for expressing myself.

Most of the time, I abuse my logical center by completely ignoring my creative side. It is okay to work in an environment that requires me to use my logical center more, such as when I work on a computer. However, I still need to balance the use of both sides of my brain so that my brain power doesn't suffer a setback.

Engaging in music, art, and writing is the easiest way to stimulate my creative center. These three activities are enough for me because when I start with one of them, my days and nights are filled with pure personal enjoyment and, more importantly, challenges to my brain, which continues to learn to do the right things.

For example, when I want to learn to draw realistic human figures, I have to learn to draw precise lines on paper. All this effort challenges my brain, which responds by increasing the number of its connections.

I don't settle for simple and ordinary solutions. I live in a society that values instant gratification, and there is nothing wrong with that thinking and attitude. However, if I settle for quick and easy solutions every time, my mind stagnates, and I feel uncreative and unmotivated.

This is why I always try to develop more creative solutions to my problems and situations. I am open to solving my problems and situations with time-tested solutions; I apply these, too, but I think of new ones simultaneously and fire up my neurons and brain cells.

I challenge my beliefs. I have my comfort zone; it is time to leave it and start learning new things. For example, when I thought sports were no longer for me, I tried Nordic walking and was seduced by it. I held back only because I feared my athletic ability would no longer be appreciated. Today, however, I challenge my beliefs.

ABOUT THE AUTHOR

Andrea Scarsi is a master of meditation who defines himself as a mystic, metaphysician, author, musician, and holistic coach when he uses his works to share a dimension of being, lifestyle, and knowledge founded on communion with the absolute.

Born in Venice, Italy, in 1955, he began practicing yoga and spiritism and experimenting with telepathy at fifteen. Following a near-death experience, he contacted alien and transdimensional entities at eighteen. At twenty-four, on his first trip to India, he found himself a vegetarian and in the world of meditation led by India and the Spiritual Master Osho. He received Swami Prem Sandesh as a new name, which he wears in specific environments.

He has often traveled, especially to India, residing for long periods in Nepal, the Philippines, Brazil, and Buddhist Southeast Asia: Japan, Thailand, Sri Lanka, Hong Kong, Laos, China, and Tibet. He has explored local places and cultures, met people, and participated in ritual and religious practices.

Over time, he delved into various meditative techniques for awakening consciousness, energy rebalancing, and personal evolution, which he practices and teaches. He studied philosophy and earned a Doctorate in Metaphysical Science and various diplomas, such as Holistic Life Coach, Reiki Grand Master, Master of Crystals, Shamanism, Meditation and Massage, and Wellness Coach. He's also into cellular nutrition and Network Marketing.

In 1991, he married Krisana, and they now live in Venice, Italy. Reach him at andrea.scarsi@yahoo.com and https://www.youtube.com/@ScarsiAndrea.

BOOKS BY ANDREA SCARSI

21 Giorni
About Osho
Answers For The Soul
Blessings!
Dead Man Walking
Extraterrestrial Channeling
Happy To Be Happy
Holistic Massage
Holistic Wellness
Home Sweet Home Staging
How To Ask A Woman Out
Imagine
Indigo Crystal Rainbow and Diamond
Journey To The Underworld
Make Your Own Vineyard
O Iguana! My Iguana!
Orchids Beauty Meditation
Overweight? No Problem!
Pearls of Wisdom
Reiki First Degree Manual
Reiki Second Degree Manual
Reiki Third Degree Manual
Romance Ain't Love Pollution
Seeds Of Enlightenment
Stop Dreaming
Swimming in The Ganges
Tarot Reading Essentials
The Art of Change
The Art of Persuasion
The Art of Worrying
The Depths Of Stillness And The Art Of Dissolving
The Foolproof Way to Fail at Online Trading
The Magic Of Money

MANTRAS BY ANDREA SCARSI (SANDESH)

Mantras Maha Mantras
The Mantra Experiment
The Mantra Way
Om Namo Supernova
Amāvasya
Lingamananda
Starship Meditations

BOOKS BY ANDREA SCARSI IN ITALIAN

21 Giorni
A Proposito di Osho
Basta Sognare
Benedizioni!
Benessere Olistico
Benvenuti ad Atlantide
Breve Storia Dei Sogni
Canalizzazioni Extraterrestri
Casa Dolce Casa Vendesi
Come Ripristino Le Capacità Del Mio Cervello
Dhyana Yoga
Dispense Reiki Primo Livello
Dispense Reiki Secondo Livello
Dispense Reiki Terzo Livello Master
Felici Di Essere Felici
Guarire il Sé Ombra
Il Lato Positronico
Il Maestro e l'Assassino
Il Modo Infallibile Per Fallire Nel Trading Online
Il Romanticismo Non è Inquinamento Emotivo
Il Segreto della Meditazione
Il Segreto della Scienza Metafisica
Il Silenzio dell'Assoluto
Immagina
Indaco Cristallo Arcobaleno e Diamante
La Cucina Vegetariana
L'Arte della Persuasione
L'Arte della Preoccupazione
L'Arte di Cambiare
L'Arte di Invitare una Donna
Le Acque sacre del Gange
Le Compatibilità Zodiacali
Le Profondità della Quiete

Lettura dei Tarocchi
Lord Shiva
Massaggio Olistico
Menando Il Can Per L'Aia
Morto Che Cammina
Notiziario Reiki
Perle di Saggezza
Risposte per l'Anima
Semi di Illuminazione
Sovrappeso? No Problem!
Transizione Vegetariana
Viaggio nel Mondo di Sotto
Zen Il Senso del Non Senso

Thank You for reading
How I restore My Brain Abilities
Dr. Andrea Scarsi

9 798301 657245